Clean Keto Diet Comfort Food
Guilt Free Indulgence For Weight Loss

Rick Elliott

Legal & Disclaimer

The information contained in this book and its contents is not designed to replace or take the place of any form of medical or professional advice; and is not meant to replace the need for independent medical, financial, legal or other professional advice or services, as may be required. The content and information in this book has been provided for educational and entertainment purposes only.

The content and information contained in this book has been compiled from sources deemed reliable, and it is accurate to the best of the Author's knowledge, information and belief. However, the Author cannot guarantee its accuracy and validity and cannot be held liable for any errors and/or omissions. Further, changes are periodically made to this book as and when needed. Where appropriate and/or necessary, you must consult a professional (including but not limited to your doctor, attorney, financial advisor or such other professional advisor) before using any of the suggested remedies, techniques, or information in this book.

Upon using the contents and information contained in this book, you agree to hold harmless the Author from and against any damages, costs, and expenses, including any legal fees potentially resulting from the application of any of the information provided by this book. This disclaimer applies to any loss, damages or injury caused by the use and application, whether directly or indirectly, of any advice or information presented, whether for breach of contract, tort, negligence, personal injury, criminal intent, or under any other cause of action.

You agree to accept all risks of using the information presented inside this book.

You agree that by continuing to read this book, where appropriate and/or necessary, you shall consult a professional (including but not limited to your doctor, attorney, or financial advisor or such other advisor as needed) before using any of the suggested remedies, techniques, or information in this book.

Legal & Disclaimer

The information contained in this book and its contents is not designed to replace or take the place of any form of medical or professional advice; and is not meant to replace the need for independent medical, financial, legal or other professional advice or services, as may be required. The content and information in this book has been provided for educational and entertainment purposes only.

The content and information contained in this book has been compiled from sources deemed reliable, and it is accurate to the best of the Author's knowledge, information and belief. However, the Author cannot guarantee its accuracy and validity and cannot be held liable for any errors and/or omissions. Further, changes are periodically made to this book as and when needed. Where appropriate and/or necessary, you must consult a professional (including but not limited to your doctor, attorney, financial advisor or such other professional advisor) before using any of the suggested remedies, techniques, or information in this book.

Upon using the contents and information contained in this book, you agree to hold harmless the Author from and against any damages, costs, and expenses, including any legal fees potentially resulting from the application of any of the information provided by this book. This disclaimer applies to any loss, damages or injury caused by the use and application, whether directly or indirectly, of any advice or information presented, whether for breach of contract, tort, negligence, personal injury, criminal intent, or under any other cause of action.

You agree to accept all risks of using the information presented inside this book.

You agree that by continuing to read this book, where appropriate and/or necessary, you shall consult a professional (including but not limited to your doctor, attorney, or financial advisor or such other advisor as needed) before using any of the suggested remedies, techniques, or information in this book.

Contents

Introduction

Adopting a Ketogenic lifestyle is not easy. We all need a little comfort food, especially to help us through tough weeks. It seems cruel to ask us to give up on warm heavy foods and snacks that brings us comfort. But there is a solution. Low Carb Keto-approved Comfort Food! And we've put together a list of Clean Keto comfort food recipes to help make sure you're staying on track with your weight goals, even when indulging in fried chicken!

Whether you're a seasoned Ketogenic dieter, or new to it, you've likely struggled with this thing – constant hunger! Every now and then you'll get a craving for something different yet worry whether you are cheating on your keto diet. There are ways of indulging without setting yourself back.

In this book, we include a collection of 30 comfort food recipes that anyone can effortlessly create meals with. They are all guaranteed to be Keto-approved diet recipes.

Chapter 1 – Keto Diet Rules

While the Keto diet is low in carbs, it's not a zero-carb diet. Getting started with the Keto diet trains your body to take only good foods that are essentially healthy and get rid of unhealthy eating habits.

According to Dr. Mike Roussell, a noted nutritionist, the Ketogenic diet allows you 50-grams intake of carbohydrates daily. No matter what you eat to curb your cravings, just don't exceed this limit. However, you need to be aware that even fruits and vegetables contain carbohydrates, making it essential to keep track of your carb intake.

You might wonder how seemingly 'unhealthy' food can be included in your keto diet? After all, even sugary food contain carbs! How can it be keto-friendly?

Load on Good Fats

Load your body with good fats including butter, coconut oil, animal fats, oil, avocados, macadamia nuts and others. It is necessary to hone your mind and body to take high amounts of good fat, low-carbs, and moderate protein content in your meals.

Limit Protein

The Keto diet is not high in protein content. General protein recommendation is 0.8 grams of protein for every pound of fat-free body weight. It is important to know your percentage of body fat. To illustrate, if your lean weight is 120 pounds, you need 96 grams (120 x 0.8 grams) of protein daily.

Not all Keto Recipes are Healthy

"Low-carb" doesn't always mean keto-approved. If you are considering going keto, make sure you do it right. Many low-carb recipes will quickly kick you out of ketosis if you aren't careful. While supposedly favored for its convenience, "dirty keto" does not bother with the quality of food or nutrients. It's full of toxins from junk food. Wouldn't you rather eat a clean healthy keto diet, detox your body, prevent disease, and lose weight?

Many so-called healthy meals are also loaded with unnecessary ingredients that could spike your blood sugar. They usually contain very high protein content — big no-no's in Keto. Stick to whole foods as much as possible and preferably homemade.

Many so-called healthy meals are also loaded with unnecessary ingredients that could spike your blood sugar. They usually contain very high protein content — big no-no's in Keto. Stick to whole foods as much as possible and preferably homemade.

Chapter 2 – The Keto Ingredients Shopping List

In Keto meal preparation, consider items that are organic and clean. These foods are nearest to their natural state and are minimally processed, thereby retaining their natural health nutrients. Such ingredients can provide you with optimal effect. Here are some of the things you need to consider in your Keto shopping list.

Sweeteners and Dairy

While it's best to avoid sweeteners on a Ketogenic diet, it remains a better alternative than sugar.

For sweeteners, stick with ones that have lower glycemic index sweeteners and there is just a small list of those used in a Keto diet. Stay away from brands with added filler ingredients like *maltodextrin* and *dextrose*. There are even others that have high glycemic sweeteners like *maltitol*. Here are some suggestions in your search for zero GI indexes.

Stevia - Liquid form is preferred. It is incredibly sweet with zero glycemic impact.

Erythritol - This is special as it passes through the body without carbs absorption.

Monk fruit - This is usually used in combination with other sweeteners for a great balancing effect.

Sucralose - A pure sweetener and must not be confused with *Splenda*. Go for the liquid version.

All these recipes don't contain dairy other than butter or ghee. If you can consume dairy, then you're alright with butter. If not, use cultured ghee as it removes most of the casein and lactose elements in butter.

Fats and Oils

Knowing the differences in fats especially when you are on a Keto diet as fat will be the primary source of your energy. In our Keto recipes, we are using ghee, coconut oil, and butter which are saturated fats. We also use monosaturated fats from olive, avocados, and nuts oil.

Saturated and monosaturated fats are more beneficial and less inflammatory to most people, although you need to watch out for your intake of seed or nut-based foods as they likewise contain the inflammatory omega 6's.

Fruits

Most fruits, especially large fruits are generally not recommended as they're high in sugar content. However, you can always manage the amount you consume. Make sure to control your portions when using them in recipes. Some fruits are used in our desserts because of their health benefits.

Examples are berries and avocados which are a powerhouse of vitamins, minerals, phytochemicals, and healthy fats. Avocados contain the least amount of sugar among fruits which makes it low-carb and Keto-friendly. Berries are excellent sources of Vitamin C, folate, potassium, and fiber.

Chocolates

You can use chocolates but be sure to choose dark chocolates (90% or more) as these have fewer carb content.

Proteins

As for sources of proteins, choose meat and eggs that are of the highest quality as these are usually grass-fed and raised in pastures. Rather than buying these products from sources located away from you, visit your nearest local farms or buy from local markets. Small-time farmers usually raised the limited quantity of these products and don't resort to using harmful chemicals that extend food shelf life.

Buy whole eggs that are organic, and when choosing nut butter, always go for the natural unsweetened nuts. Also, choose the fattier version such as almond butter and macadamia nut butter. Peanuts have high omega 6's content so be careful not to over consume.

Nuts and Seed Flours

These are great substitutes for regular flour. Almond flour and seeds as in flaxseed meal must be eaten in moderation. Also, try mixing multiple flours to enhance texture in baking. Experimenting with your cooking can lead to much lower net carbs counts in dishes. Note that different flours can act in relatively different ways like the amount of coconut flour is equivalent to half of the amount of the almond flour. This is because coconut flour tends to be more absorptive and requires more liquid.

Chapter 3 – 30 Keto Food Recipes

#1 – Tomatoes with Beans and Sausage

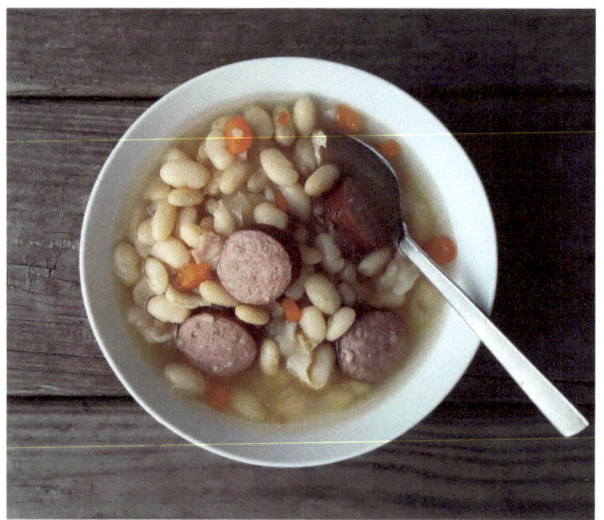

Ingredients

- 2 Italian sausages

- 1 Onion

- 2 Cloves of Garlic

- 1 tbsp. Olive oil

- 1/2 tsp. Basil (dried)

- 1/2 tsp. Oregano (dried)

- 28-oz. can Crushed tomatoes

- A pinch of Red pepper flakes

- Ground pepper (freshly cracked)

- 2 15-oz. cans of White Beans

- Sea salt to taste

Directions

1. Add olive oil in a cooking pot and fry sausages in medium-low heat until brown. Once cooked, cut sausages into slices and return to pot.

2. Sauté with garlic and onions until sausages become evenly browned and later transparent. While stirring, scrape the bits of sausages off the bottom of the pot. Add crushed tomatoes, add spices and seasonings.

3. Meanwhile, rinse white beans with water and drain. Add beans to the pot along with chopped spinach. Stir and allow to heat through for about 10 minutes. Add salt to taste. Simmer longer to reduce the amount of liquid if you want to have a thicker consistency and serve hot with crusty bread.

Nutritional Value: Calories – 145.6; Net Carbs – 0.4 grams; Protein – 16.7 grams; Fat – 8.2 grams

#2 - Bacon & Guacamole Bombs

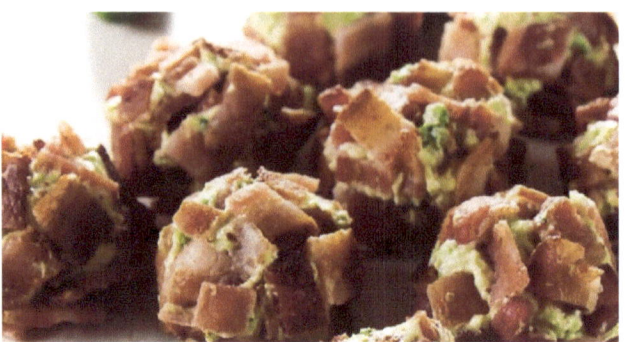

Ingredients

- 4 Large bacon slices

- 1/2 Large avocado (Pitted and peeled)

- 1/4 cup Butter (Softened at room temperature)

- 2 cloves Garlic (Crushed)

- 1 Small chili pepper (Finely chopped)

- 1/2 Small white onion (Diced)

- 1-2 tbsp. Cilantro (Freshly chopped)

- 1 tbsp Fresh lime juice

- 1/4 tsp. Salt

- Freshly ground black pepper

Directions

1. Preheat oven to 375°F.

2. Line a baking sheet with parchment paper. Put the bacon strips, observing space in between so they would crisp up.

3. Cook the bacon for about 10-15 minutes or until golden brown. Remove from the oven and set aside to cool down.

4. While waiting for the bacon, mix the avocado, garlic, butter, chili pepper, cilantro, and lime juice in a bowl. Season with salt and pepper.

5. Using a fork or potato masher, mash the avocado together with the other ingredients until they're well combined. Add the onions and the bacon grease from the tray. Mix well.

6. Cover the bowl with foil and refrigerate for 20 minutes to half an hour. Meanwhile, crumble the bacon into bits.

7. Once the refrigeration time is up, get the guacamole mixture. Using an ice cream scoop or spoon, make 6 guacamole balls. Roll each ball in bacon bits and place in serving plate.

8. Serve immediately or store in an air-tight container then refrigerate for up to 5 days.

Nutritional Value: Calories- 156; Net Carbs- 1.4 grams; Protein- 3.4 grams; Fat- 15.2 grams

#3 – Bacon Wrapped Meatballs

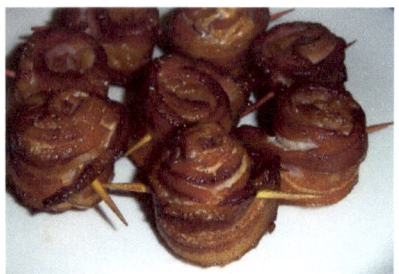

Ingredients

- 18 Bacon slices (Halved)

- 1 lb. Ground beef

- 1 lb. Ground pork

- ¼ cup Grated Parmesan

- 1 Egg (Beaten)

- 1 tsp. Onion powder

- 1 tbsp. Italian seasoning

- Low-carb barbecue sauce

- Salt

- Black pepper

- Chopped parsley (For garnish, optional)

-

Directions

1. Preheat the oven to 350°F.

2. In a large mixing bowl, combine the beef, pork, egg, onion powder, Italian seasoning, salt, pepper, and Parmesan. Mix well.

3. Line a baking sheet with aluminum foil and put a baking rack inside (grease with non-stick spray if it's not the non-stick kind).

4. Make 36 small meatballs and wrap each up with bacon. Place each into the rack with the seam side down. Make sure to put enough space between meatballs.

5. Bake for about 15 minutes. Get the sheet from the oven and brush the meatballs with the barbecue sauce.

6. Bake again for another 15 minutes or until the meatballs are cooked through.

7. Let them cool for a bit. Serve with parsley if desired and extra barbecue sauce for dipping.

Nutritional Value: Calories- 669; Net Carbs- 2 grams; Protein- 35 grams; Fat- 56 grams

#4 – Chicken Zoodle Soup

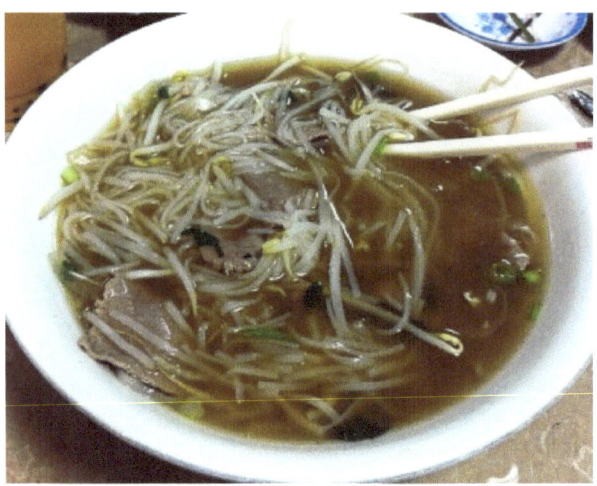

Ingredients

- 3 pcs. Medium-sized zucchini (spiraled)

- 2 tbs. Olive oil

- 1 lb. Chicken breasts (skinless, deboned, and cut into chunks)

- 3 carrots (diced)

- 3 Cloves of garlic (minced)

- 1 Onion (diced_

- 2 Celery stalks (sliced)

- Freshly ground black pepper

- 4 cups Chicken stock

- 2 tbsp. Lemon juice extract

- ¼ tsp. Dried rosemary

- 1 Bay leaf

- ½ tsp. Dried thyme

- 2 tbsp. Fresh parsley leaves (chopped)

- 1 sprig of fresh rosemary

Directions

1. Pour a tablespoon of olive oil in a large stockpot. Heat it over medium heat.

2. In a mixing bowl, season chicken with salt and pepper and transfer it to the stockpot. Allow it to cook until it turns golden brown and then set aside.

3. Pour remaining oil into the pot and sauté carrots and celery with garlic and onions. Cook until the carrots are tender before stirring in thyme and rosemary for about an hour.

4. Add chicken stock with 2 cups of water along with the bay leaf. Bring to a boil and stir in chicken and zucchini noodles. Allow it to simmer by reducing heat until zucchini becomes tender. This takes about 3 minutes. Add lemon extract and season with salt and pepper.

5. Serve while warm and garnish with fresh parsley and rosemary.

Nutritional Value: Calories – 317; Net Carbs – 28 grams; Protein – 42 grams; Fat – 7 grams

#5 – Brownie Fudge

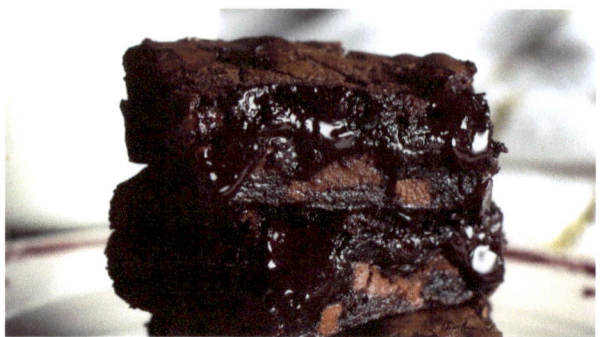

Ingredients

- 1/4 tsp. Baking soda

- 5 tbsp. Cacao powder

- 2 tsp. Vanilla extract

- 2 tbsp. Melted Butter (Coconut oil or ghee)

- 3/4 cup Coconut butter (melted)

- 1 Large egg

- 1/3 cup Full-fat Coconut milk cream

- 3/4 cup Sweetener (granulated)

- 1/2 tsp. Vanilla bean powder

- 1/4 tsp. Sea salt

Directions

1. Combine cocoa powder, vanilla bean powder, baking soda, salt, the sweetener in a mixing bowl and then set aside for later use.

2. In another bowl, put the melted coconut cream, butter, and coconut milk cream. Beat to blend until smooth.

3. Combine the dry and wet ingredients and mix thoroughly by beating until there are no signs of lumps evident.

4. Spread the mixture in a prepared pan, greased or lined with parchment paper.

5. Bake at 350 degrees Fahrenheit for 20-25 minutes until edges get brownish in color. The center may not yet be well done but it's alright at this point.

6. Allow the pan to cool before storing it in the refrigerator.

7. Serve when needed.

Note: You can melt the coconut cream or butter by placing it in a jar and place it over boiling water until inside is melted.

Nutritional Value: Calories –172; Net Carbs – 9 grams; Protein – 4 grams; Fat – 16 grams

#6 – Brussels Sprouts Chips

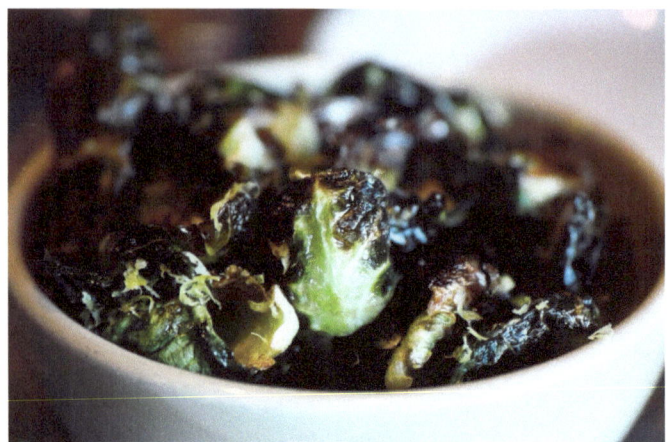

Ingredients

- 1 lb. Brussels sprouts (Washed and dried)

- 2 tbsp. Extra virgin olive oil

- 1 tsp. Kosher salt

- Paprika (Optional)

- Cumin (Optional)

Directions

1. . Preheat the oven to 400°F.

2. While at it, prepare the Brussels sprouts. Trim the base and peel off the excess or any tough leaves until you get a tight head. If you want, cut off the exposed stalk some more. Put to a bowl when done. Repeat this step to each sprout.

3. Pour some oil to the sprouts and toss. Using your clean hands, rub the oil to each piece, making sure that all of them are well-coated. Season with salt and toss again.

4. Get a baking sheet or two (to accommodate all the sprouts) and spread the sprouts. Make sure that they don't stack up on each other and they have enough space apart. This allows the sprouts to really crisp up.

5. Bake for 10-15 minutes or until achieve a deep brown color. Once done, remove from oven and let them cool for a bit.

6. Season with salt and spices (paprika and cumin) if you like and serve.

Nutritional Value: Calories – 256; Net Carbs – 3 grams; Protein – 13 grams; Fat – 20 grams

#7 – Blueberry-Chocolate Clusters

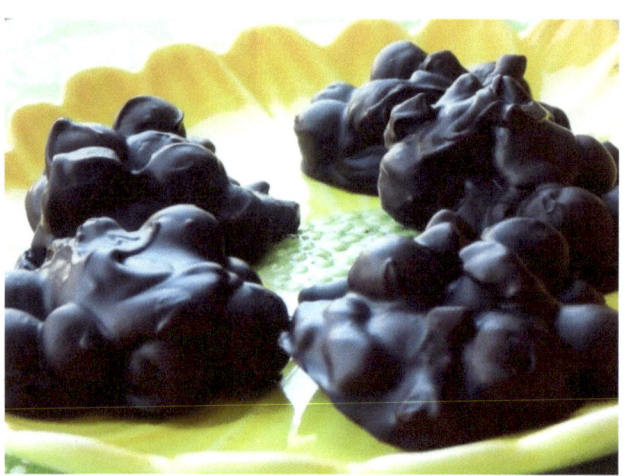

Ingredients

- 2 cups Blueberries

- 1 ½ cups Semi-sweet chocolate chips (melted)

- Flaky sea salt (for garnish)

- 1 tbsp. Coconut oil

Directions

1. Prepare baking sheet lined with parchment paper.

2. Melt chocolate chips in a medium-size bowl added with coconut oil.

3. Drop a little amount of the chocolate mixture on the parchment and place 3 blueberries on top of it. Drizzle it with chocolate mixture and sprinkle with sea salt.

4. Repeat the process until you have filled up the baking sheet. Provide enough space in between.

5. Freeze to set for about 10 minutes before serving.

Nutritional Value: Calories – 56; Net Carbs – 5 grams; Protein – 1.7 grams; Fat – 3 grams

#8 – Cheese and Bacon Stuffed Tomatoes

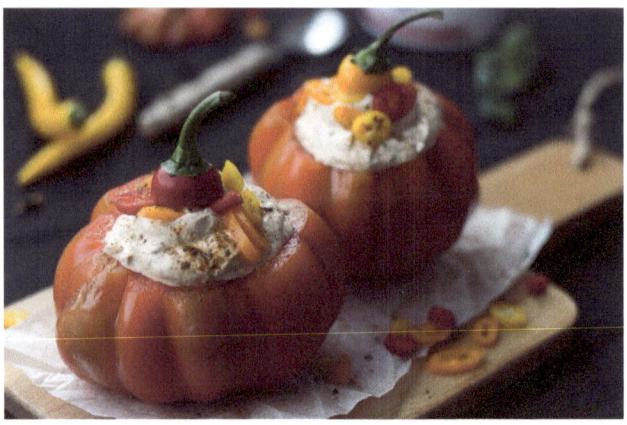

Ingredients

- 6 Large tomatoes (pitted)

- 4 Slices bacon (Cooked and crumbled)

- 1/2 cup Shredded cheddar cheese (Plus extra for topping)

- 4 oz. Cream cheese

- 2 tbsp. Green onions (Sliced)

- 1/2 tsp. Garlic powder

- 1 tsp. Worcestershire sauce

- Chopped cilantro (For garnish, optional)

Directions

1. Preheat oven to 400° F.

2. Grease a cookie sheet using non-stick cooking spray and set aside.

3. In a small mixing bowl, combine bacon, cheddar, cream cheese, green onions, garlic powder, and Worcestershire sauce together. You can use a whisk or electric mixer to achieve a smooth consistency.

4. Fill tomatoes with the bacon and cheese mixture and line them in the cookie sheet. Sprinkle with extra cheddar and put into the oven.

5. Bake for 10-12 minutes until tomatoes are softened and the cheese is bubbly.

6. Take off from the oven and let them cool for a bit. Sprinkle with cilantro if desired before serving.

Nutritional Value: Calories - 87; Net Carbs- 1 gram; Protein- 2 grams; Fat- 7 grams

#9 – Cheesy Pepperoni Chips

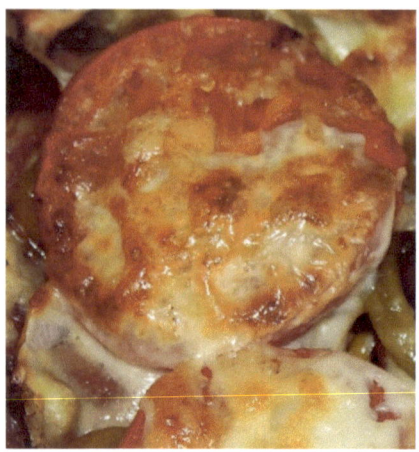

Ingredients

- 6 oz. Pepperoni slices

- oz. Mozzarella cheese (Shredded)

- Marinara sauce (For dipping, optional)

Directions

1. Preheat oven to 400°F.

2. Prepare 2-3 cookie sheets.

3. Assemble the pepperoni slices in groups of four. Make the Pepperoni sides by the center of the group to overlap with each other.

4. Bake them for about 5 minutes until they're semi-crispy. Just arrange them back together if they somehow move out of place.

5. Add cheese on top and bring them back to the oven. Bake for another 3 minutes or until the Pepperoni has crisp up.

6.   Transfer then chips on a plate with paper towels. This will remove the excess oil. Let them sit for about 3-4 minutes or until they're completely cool. If desired, serve with marinara sauce.

Nutritional Value: Calories – 61.29; Net Carbs- 0.16 grams; Protein- 3 grams; Fat- 5.3 grams

#10 – Omelette Waffle

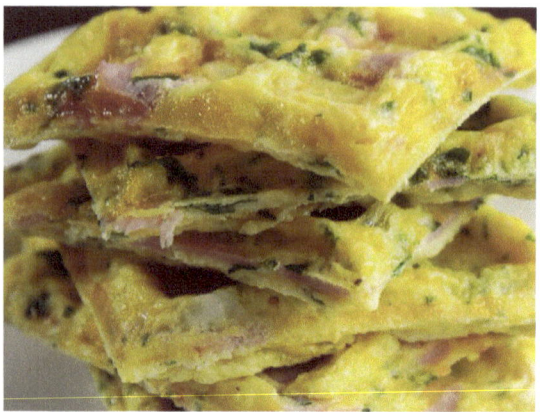

Ingredients

- 1 tbsp. of Mozzarella cheese (shredded)

- 1 tbsp. Red pepper (finely chopped)

- 1 tbsp. Broccoli (finely chopped)

- 1 tbsp. of sausage (finely sliced)

- 2 tsp. Palm oil

Directions

1. Preheat waffle iron and spray with palm oil on both sides (top and bottom). In a mixing bowl, combine milk and egg and whisk to form the batter. Once the waffle molder is hot, pour the batter carefully. See to it that it is filled up just below the top level. Leave enough space to allow the waffle to rise. Filling up all the space will cause a leak on the sides, messing up your dish.

2. Cook in the same process until all batter is used up.

Nutritional Value: Calories – 317; Net Carbs – 1.63 grams; Protein – 7.67 grams; Fat – 30.92 grams

#11 – Simple Egg Salad with Bacon and Lettuce

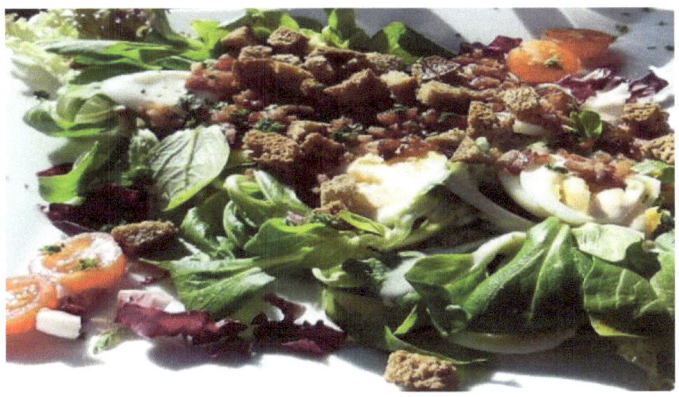

Ingredients

- 6 eggs

- 2 tbsp. of mayonnaise

- 1 tsp. of lemon juice

- 1 tsp. of Dijon mustard

- ¼ tsp. of lite salt

- Kosher salt

- Pepper

- 4 Romaine lettuce leaves

- 2 slices of bacon

Directions

1. Boil the eggs for about 10 minutes, remove from heat and set aside to cool

2. Peel the eggs and process in a food processor until they're chopped.

3. Add the mayonnaise, lemon juice, mustard, pepper plus the lite and kosher salts

4. Serve with lettuce leaves and bacon.

Nutritional Value: Calories – 262 calories, 21g fat, 16g protein, 1g net carbohydrates

#12 – Cookie Dough Fat Bomb

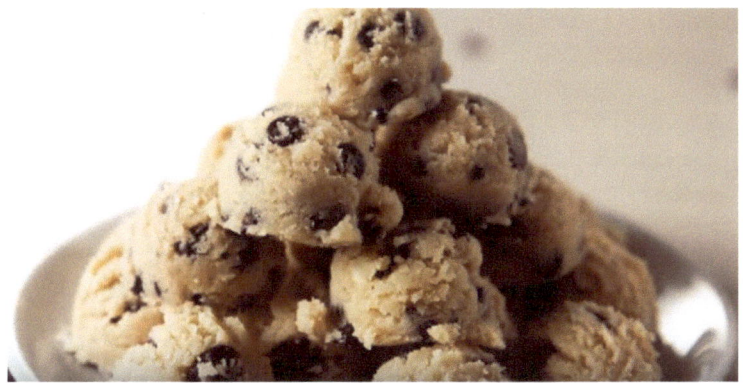

Ingredients

- ½ cup Coconut oil (melted)

- ¼ cup Dark chocolate (finely chopped)

- ¾ cup Almond Flour

- 1 tbsp. Maple syrup

- ¼ cup Almond butter

- 1/2 tsp. Vanilla extract

- 1/2 tsp. Kosher salt

Directions

1. In a mixing bowl, combine coconut oil, almond butter, maple syrup, and almond flour. Mix all ingredients thoroughly using a mixer. Add in dark chocolate. Cover the bowl with a plastic wrap and keep in the fridge for 15-20 minutes until slightly firm.

2. When the mixture hardens, scoop into small balls using a cookie scoop. You can store this in the refrigerator for up to a month.

Nutritional Value: Calories –209; Carbs – 6.7 grams; Protein – 3.4 grams; Fat – 19.9 grams

#13 – Easy Avocado Dessert

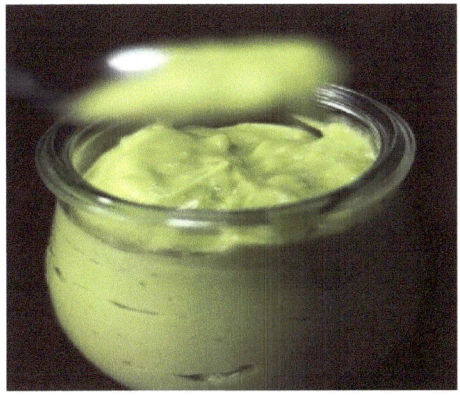

Ingredients

- 1.5 oz. Heavy cream

- 2 small Avocados (ripe)

- Sweetener to taste

Directions

1. Peel avocados skin and remove pits.

2. Spoon avocado flesh into a bowl.

3. Add Sweetener

4. Mash avocado using the back of a spoon

5. Add heavy cream and keep in the refrigerator to chill for about an hour.

Nutritional Value: Calories –146; Net Carbs – 18.3 grams; Protein – 2 grams; Fat – 8 grams

#14 – Easy Keto Brownies

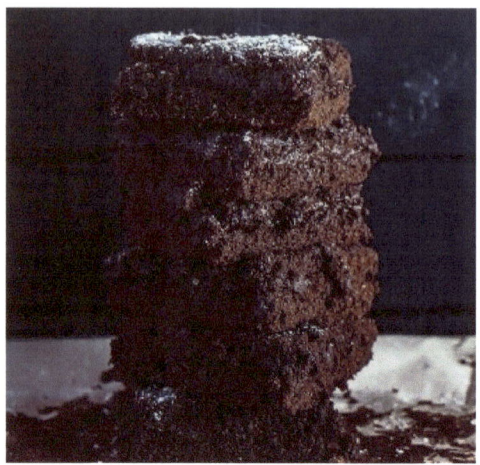

Ingredients

- 1/2 cup Butter

- 2 Eggs (large)

- 2 Egg yolks

- 1/2 cup Unsweetened dark chocolate chips

- 2 tbsp. Coconut flour

- 1/4 cup Almond milk

- 1 tsp. Vanilla extract

- 2 tbsp. Unsweetened cocoa powder

- 1/2 tsp. Baking powder

- 2 tbsp. Erythritol

- 1 shot Espresso (cold)

- Pinch of salt

Directions

1. Preheat oven to 375 degrees Fahrenheit.

2. Melt chocolate chips and butter in the microwave on high heat for 1-2 minutes. Stir to blend.

3. Add vanilla, espresso, and erythritol to chocolate mixture and stir to combine.

4. Add eggs and egg yolks in a separate bowl and beat lightly. Slowly add this egg mixture into your chocolate mixture while whisking to avoid cooking the eggs.

5. Add coconut flour, salt, baking powder, and cocoa powder. Mix thoroughly to blend all ingredients.

6. Transfer batter into a well-greased 8x8-inch brownie pan or lined with parchment paper. Spread the batter evenly.

7. Bake for 8-9 minutes. Take the cooked brownie out of the oven and leave to cool. Cut and serve. Make sure that your brownie has completely cooled down lest it crumbles once you slice.

Nutritional Value: Calories – 158; Net Carbs – 9.01 grams; Protein – 3.84 grams; Fat – 14.29 grams

#15 - Easy Orange Cake Balls

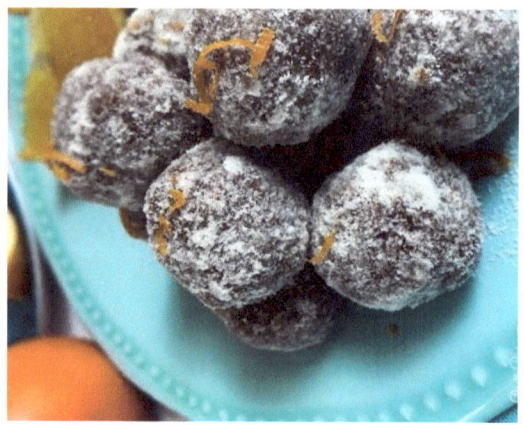

Ingredients

- 2/3 cup Almond butter

- 1/3 cup Coconut flour + more for rolling

- Orange zest

- 1/4 cup Orange juice

- 35 drops Stevia to taste

- 1/2 tsp. Vanilla extract

- Pinch of Himalayan salt

Directions

1. Combine all ingredients in a mixing bowl and mix well.

2. If the mixture turns too dry, add a small amount of orange juice or drizzle with avocado oil to adjust. Add coconut flour when too wet. Add sweetener to suit your taste.

3. Using a cookie scoop, make balls and use your hands to smoothen them.

4. Roll balls lightly over coconut flour to cover. If you want to have them firmer, chill for about 10 minutes in the refrigerator.

Nutritional Value: Calories – 218.8; Net Carbs – 037.4 grams; Protein – 2.2 grams; Fat - 3.1 grams

#16 – Crispy Pork Belly Bites

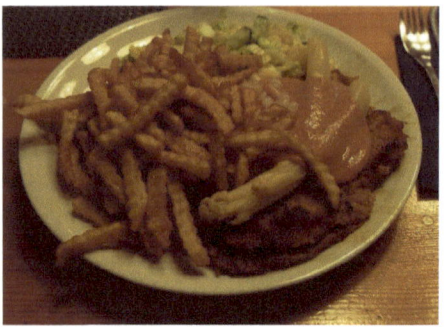

Ingredients

- 10.5 oz. Thin pork belly strips

- 1.76 oz. Blue cheese

- 4 tbsp. Heavy whipping cream

- 1 tbsp. Butter

- ¼ Large white onion (Diced)

- 1 tsp. Salt

- Pepper

Directions

1. Preheat oven to 475°F.

2. Meanwhile, rub some salt to the pork belly strips, making sure that they're coated with thin layer of salt. Put them in an oven dish.

3. Bake the pork strips for about 30-45 minutes, periodically monitoring them. Once they turn into golden brown, they're already done.

4. While baking the pork, place a pan over medium heat. Put the butter and cook the onions until they're caramelized. They should turn translucent with a sweet flavor.

5. Once the onion is done, add the whipping cream. Warm it through.

6. Once the cream is warmed through, add the blue cheese. Break the cheese so it can easily melt.

7. When the cheese has completely melted, adjust heat to high for 1-2 minutes. Turn off the heat and immediately transfer the cheese mixture into a dish.

8. Remove the pork from the oven and let it cool on a plate with paper towel. Cut them into bite-size pieces. Transfer to a plate and serve with cheese dip on the side.

Nutritional Value: Calories – 448; Net Carbs- 1.9 grams; Protein- 19.61 grams; Fat- 40.56 grams

#17 – Fried Cauliflower Rice

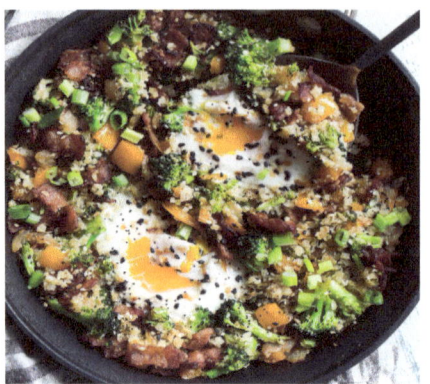

Ingredients

- 4 Slices nitrate free bacon cut into bite size pieces {Sugar free for Whole30}

- 2 Tbsp cooking fat divided (you can use the rendered bacon fat)

- 8 oz riced cauliflower

- 1 small onion diced

- 1 small red bell pepper diced

- 6 oz broccoli florets cut into bite size pieces

- 2 tsp coconut aminos

- Sea salt and pepper to taste

- 3 large eggs Or one per person

- Trader Joe's everything bagel seasoning **

- Thinly sliced green onion for garnish

Directions

1. Heat a skillet over medium high heat. Add the bacon pieces and cook until crisp, stirring to even brown. Once done, remove to a plate, set aside.

2. If using the rendered bacon fat for cooking, save 2 Tbsp and leave about 1 Tbsp in the skillet. If not, discard bacon fat and add 1 Tbsp of preferred fat to skillet.

3. Lower heat to medium and add the onions, stir to coat. Cook until softened, then add pepper and continue to cook another minute, stirring.

4. Add another Tbsp cooking fat along with the broccoli and stir to coat. Sprinkle with salt, pepper and seasoning. Cover skillet for 30 seconds to soften broccoli.

5. Uncover skillet and add the bacon, cauliflower rice, and coconut aminos. Stir to fully coat cauliflower rice with the other veggies and bacon. Cook, stirring occasionally for 45-60 seconds or until softened.

6. Lower the heat to low and create 2 grooves for the eggs. Add a bit of fat to each groove and crack an egg in each one. Sprinkle with salt, pepper, and seasoning of choice, then cover the skillet and cook about 2 minutes, or until eggs are cooked to preference.

7. Remove from heat and garnish with thinly sliced scallions if desired.

Nutritional Value: Calories- 327; Net Carbs- 7.93 grams; Protein- 12 grams; Fat- 25 grams

#18 – Keto Chocolate Cake Less the Flour

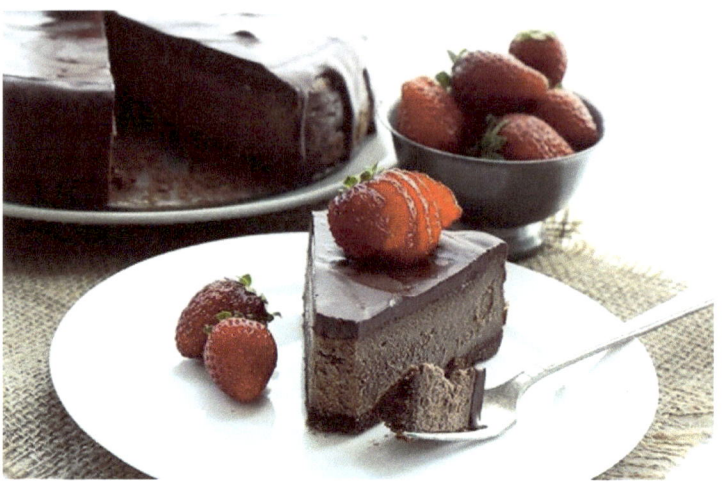

Ingredients

- 4 Eggs, large

- 12 oz. Unsweetened baking chocolate

- 2/3 cup Butter or ghee (cut into pieces - tablespoon-size)

- 1/3 cup Water

- 1/2 cup Low-carb sweetener

- Boiling water

- 1/4 teaspoon salt

Directions

1. Line a 9-inch Springform pan with parchment paper.

2. In a small pot, boil water over medium heat. Add salt and sweetener and let boil under fully dissolved.

3. In a double boiler, melt the baking chocolate. You may also use a microwave as an alternative.

4. In a large bowl, add the melted chocolate and butter and then mix using an electric mixer. Add the sweetened mixture and continue beating.

5. Gradually add the eggs one after the other. Beat well after each addition.

6. Pour the mixture into the Springform pan and cover it well with foil.

7. Insert the Springform pan inside a larger cake pan and pour boiling water to about an inch deep.

8. Bake for about 45 minutes at 360 degrees Fahrenheit. When cooked, remove and allow cooling on a wire rack.

9. Chill the cake inside the fridge overnight.

10. Remove the cake from the Springform pan and serve.

Nutritional Value: Calories – 295; Net Carbs – 8grams; Protein – 6 grams; Fat – 26grams

#19 – Keto Coconut Mocha Donuts

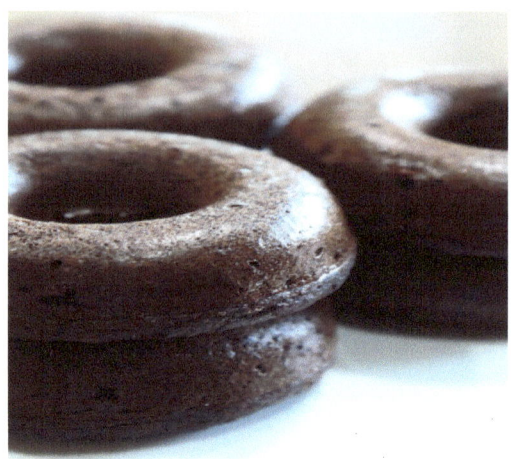

Ingredients

- 4 Eggs

- 1/3 cup Coconut or almond milk (unsweetened)

- 1/3 cup Coconut Flour

- 3 tbsp. Cocoa powder (unsweetened)

- 1/2 tsp. baking soda

- 1/4 cup coconut oil

- 1 tbsp. Liquid Stevia

- 1/2 tsp. Instant coffee granules

- 1/2 tsp. Baking powder

Directions

1. Place all ingredients in a mixing bowl and mix to blend.

2. Preheat the oven to 350 degrees Fahrenheit.

3. Pour mixture into a greased doughnut pan and bake for 20 minutes.

4. Place on a cooling rack and allow cooling.

5. Serve and enjoy!

Nutritional Value: Calories – 161; Net Carbs – 5 grams; Protein – 5 grams; Fat – 14 grams

#20 – Southern Fried Chicken with Baby Spinach

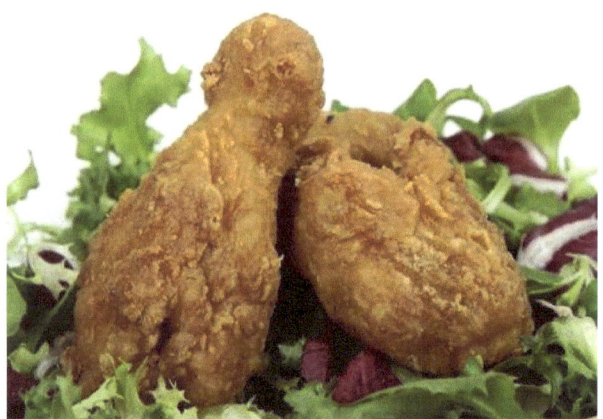

Ingredients

- 5 lbs. of chicken leg quarters

- 1 cup of coconut flour

- 1 tsp. of paprika

- 1 tsp. of garlic powder

- 1 tsp. of salt

- 1 tsp. of pepper

- Oil, for frying

Directions

1. Combine the chicken, garlic powder, paprika, salt and pepper in a large bowl. Massage the spices to the chicken until it's well coated. Cover the bowl and refrigerate for 2 hours (or overnight if you want it to be more flavorful).

2. To cook, add the coconut flour and mix to coat well. Heat 2-inch deep oil in a large skillet (or deep fryer) to 375°F.

3. Cook the chicken in batches for 8 minutes per side or until it's golden brown. If you want them to be crisp, don't overcrowd your pan. Use a meat thermometer to know if the internal temperature reaches 165°F. Alternatively, you can cut the meat to make sure that it's no longer pink.

4. Serve with 2 cups of raw baby spinach together dressed with 1 tbsp. of sugar- free ranch dressing.

Nutritional Value:

- Southern Fried Chicken: 425 calories, 32g fat, 34g protein, 1g net carbohydrates
- •Baby Spinach: 14 calories, 0g fat, 2g protein, 1g net carbohydrates
- •Ranch Dressing: 70 calories, 7g fat, 0g protein, 1g net carbohydrates

#21 – Keto Low-Carb Pumpkin

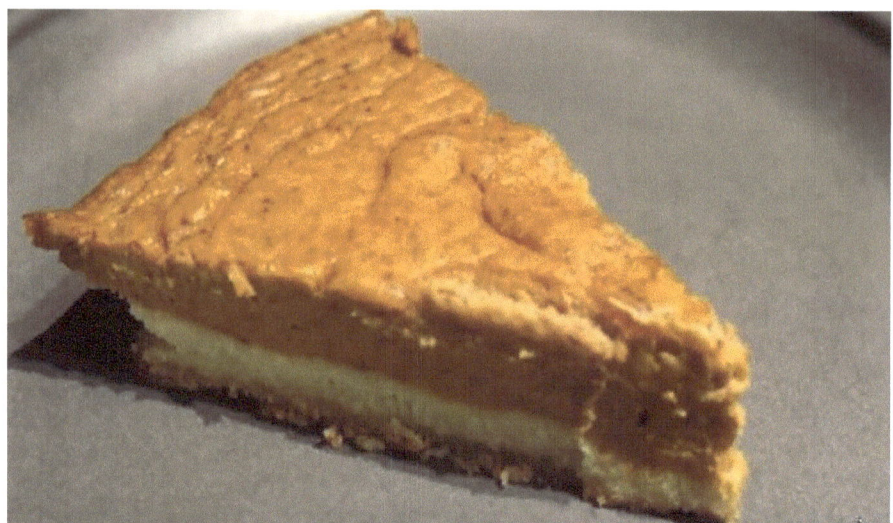

Ingredients

- 1 - 15-oz. Pumpkin puree (unsweetened)

- 2 tbsp. Pumpkin pie spice

- ¾ cup Heavy cream

- 12 oz. Cream cheese (softened)

- 1/2 cup Erythritol

- 2 tbsp. Vanilla extract (pure)

Directions

1. Combine pumpkin puree and cream cheese in a large mixing bowl. Mix thoroughly using a hand mixer until mixture turns smooth and creamy. Make sure no visible lumps are left.

2. Add vanilla extract, heavy cream, and pumpkin pie spice. Mix well to blend all ingredients completely.

3.   Leave in the refrigerator to cool before serving.

Nutritional Value: Calories – 215; Net Carbs – 3 grams; Protein – 3 grams; Fat –
18 grams

#22 – Keto Mozzarella Cheese Sticks

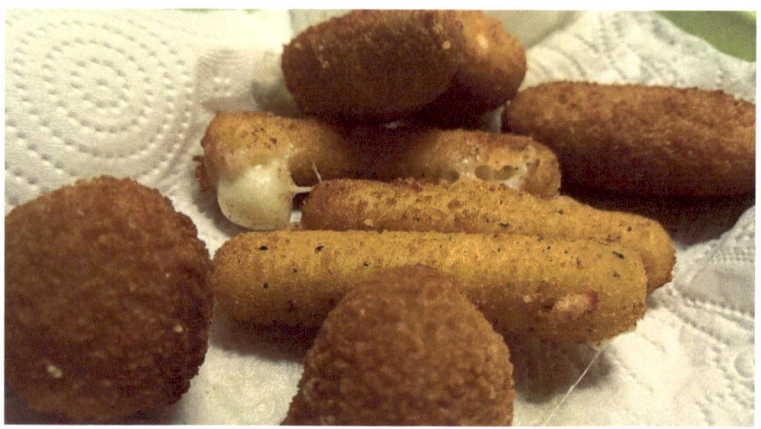

Ingredients

- 8 Regular mozzarella cheese sticks

- 1/2 cup Grated parmesan cheese

- 1 Large egg

- 1/4 cup Almond Flour

- 1 tsp. Italian Seasoning

- 1 tsp. Garlic powder

- 1/4 tsp. Ground rosemary

Directions

1. Remove cheese sticks from wrapper and set aside.

2. Whisk the egg in a shallow bowl, making sure that the white and yolk are completely combined.

3. Combine the parmesan cheese, almond flour, garlic powder, Italian seasoning, and rosemary together in another bowl. Mix well and leave no lumps.

4. Roll each cheese stick into the whisked egg first then into the flour mixture. Repeat this step once again until all sticks are well coated.

5. Line them on a cookie sheet lined with parchment paper and freeze completely.

6. After freezing, bake in a preheated oven (400°F) for about 4-5 minutes, turning them halfway through for even cooking.

Nutritional Value: Calories – 62; Net Carbs- 2 grams; Protein- 4 grams; Fat- 4 grams

#23 – Pistachio Toffee Cups

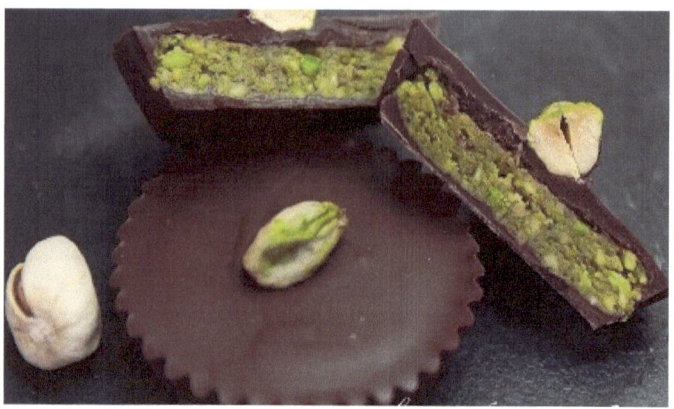

Ingredients

- 5 oz. Salted milk chocolate

- 3 tbsp. and 2 tsp. Erythritol (granulated sweetener)

- 3 tbsp. Butter (unsalted)

- ½ oz. Raw pistachios, chopped

- 1/2 tsp. Vanilla extract

- Salt to taste

Directions

1. Melt half of the chocolate in a double boiler, stirring frequently to prevent chocolates from sticking to the bottom of the pan. Save half of the chocolate for later use.

2. Line a cupcake pan with cupcake liners (you may use a silicone candy mold if you want) and brush the bottom and sides with melted chocolates. Put the mold in the refrigerator for about ten minutes for the chocolate to set.

3. In a small mixing bowl, combine butter and sweetener and melt it over low heat in a microwave for 10 seconds. As the mixture turns light brown in color, remove from the microwave and add an additional 2 teaspoons of sweetener, vanilla extract, and pistachios. Stir to mix.

4. Quickly fill two-thirds of the cupcake molds with the toffee mixture. Work fast as the mixture hardens quickly as it gets cold. Melt what remains of the chocolate and cover the molds with it to smoothen. Keep candies on the fridge for an hour or more to chill. Serve when needed.

Nutritional Value: Calories – 161; Net Carbs – 5 grams; Protein – 5 grams; Fat – 14 grams

#24 – Simple Caprese Salad

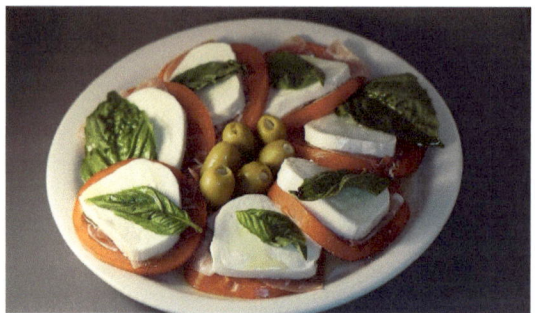

Ingredients

- 6 oz. Fresh mozzarella cheese

- 1 Large tomato

- ¼ cup Fresh Basil (Chopped)

- 3 tbsp. Olive oil

- Salt

- Pepper

Directions

1. Process the basil and olive oil in a food processor to make a paste.

2. Cut the tomato into quarter-inch slices (about 6 slices).

3. Divide the mozzarella into 1-ounce slices.

4. Arrange the salad by layering the tomato (bottom), mozzarella, and basil paste (center of mozzarella).

5. Season it with salt and pepper. Drizzle with oil.

Nutritional Value: Calories – 451; Net Carbs- 4.34 grams; Protein- 19.75 grams; Fat- 39.46 grams

#25 – Pistachio Toffee Cups

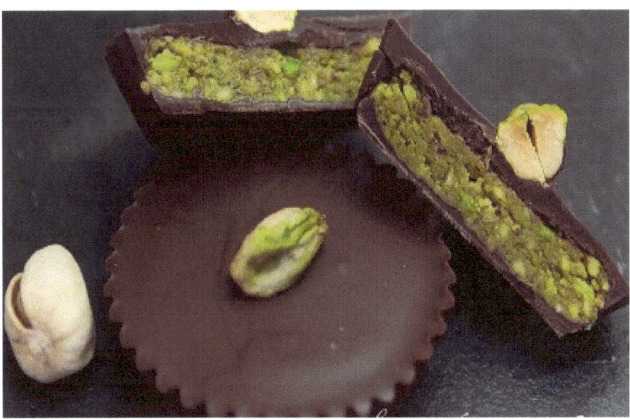

Ingredients

- 5 oz. Salted milk chocolate

- 3 tbsp. and 2 tsp. Erythritol (granulated sweetener)

- 3 tbsp. Butter (unsalted)

- ½ oz. Raw pistachios, chopped

- 1/2 tsp. Vanilla extract

- Salt to taste

Directions

1. Melt half of the chocolate in a double boiler, stirring frequently to prevent chocolates from sticking to the bottom of the pan. Save half of the chocolate for later use.

2. Line a cupcake pan with cupcake liners (you may use a silicone candy mold if you want) and brush the bottom and sides with melted chocolates. Put the mold in the refrigerator for about ten minutes for the chocolate to set.

3. In a small mixing bowl, combine butter and sweetener and melt it over low heat in a microwave for 10 seconds. As the mixture turns light brown in color, remove from the microwave and add an additional 2 teaspoons of sweetener, vanilla extract, and pistachios. Stir to mix.

4. Quickly fill two-thirds of the cupcake molds with the toffee mixture. Work fast as the mixture hardens quickly as it gets cold. Melt what remains of the chocolate and cover the molds with it to smoothen. Keep candies on the fridge for an hour or more to chill. Serve when needed.

Nutritional Value: Calories – 161; Net Carbs – 5 grams; Protein – 5 grams; Fat – 14 grams

#26 – Salmon Lettuce Cups with Lemon-Basil Spread

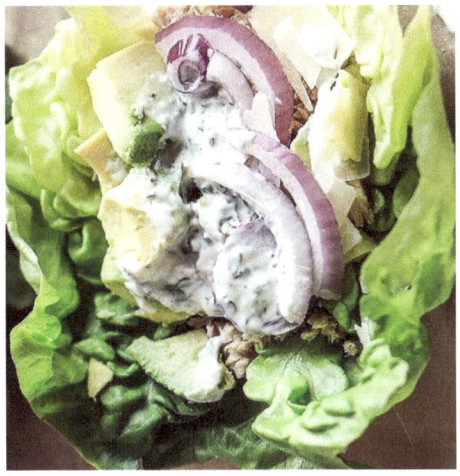

Ingredients

- 5 oz. can Pink salmon (drained)

- 2 leaves of Boston lettuce (washed)

- ½ Medium avocados (cubed)

- ¼ oz. Fresh basil (finely chopped)

- 4 tbsp. Mayonnaise

- 2 tbsp. Parmesan cheese (shaved)

- 1 tsp. Lemon juice

- ½ tsp. Garlic powder

- 1 oz. Red onion (sliced)

Directions

1. To make the spread, incorporate the basil, garlic, and lemon juice in a mixing bowl. Mix well to completely coat the basil with seasonings.

2. Add the mayo and stir. Set aside.

3. Get the lettuce leaves and fill each with a half cup of salmon. Top with avocado and onions.

4. Spoon about 2 tablespoons of mayo spread on top of each cup. Garnish with Parmesan cheese. You can also divide the mayo spread between two portions to serve as a dip.

Nutritional Value: Calories –373.5; Net Carbs- 2.83 grams; Protein- 19.63 grams; Fat- 30.87 grams

#27 – Strawberry in Chocolate Cubes

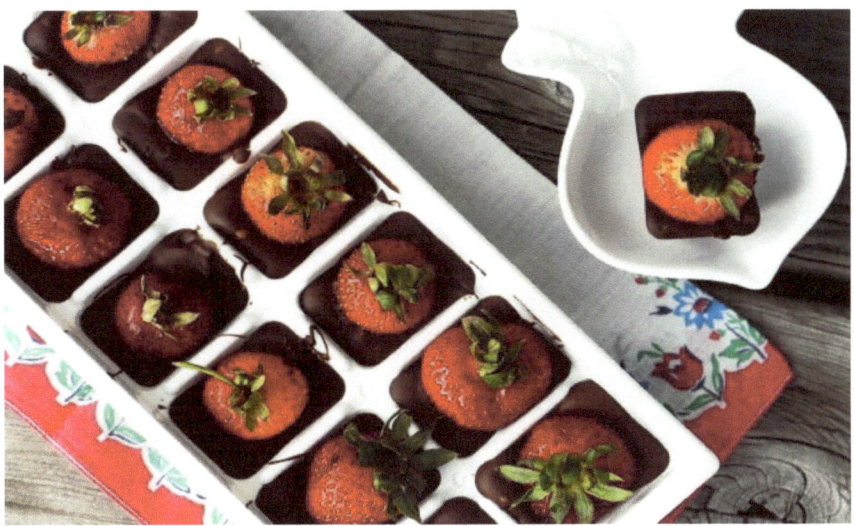

Ingredients

- 16 Strawberries (fresh and with stems)

- 2 cups Chocolate chips

- 2 tbsp. Coconut oil

Directions

1. Mix melted chocolates and coconut oil in a medium-sized bowl.

2. Drop a dollop of the chocolate mixture to fill the bottom of each cube mold in an ice tray. Place a strawberry on top of each with stem pointing upward. Spoon remaining mixture and drop over each mold.

3. Freeze for about 4-5 hours to solidify before serving.

Nutritional Value: Calories – 175; Net Carbs – 5grams; Protein – 3 grams; Fat – 9 grams

#28 – Herb-Roasted Pork Loin

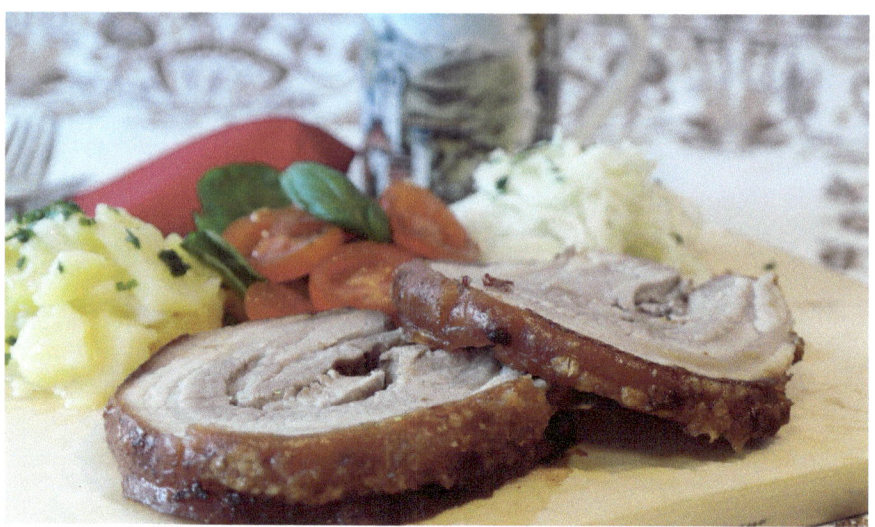

Ingredients

- 1 1/2 Pork loin

- 1 tsp. Dried basil

- 2 cloves of garlic (minced)

- 1 tsp. Dried rosemary

- 10 Fresh crack pepper

- 2 tbsp. Olive oil

- Salt to taste

Directions

1. Start by preheating the oven to 425 degrees Fahrenheit. Add seasonings, herbs, and spices in a food processor and pulse. Transfer the mixture to a mixing bowl and add oil. Toss to blend.

2. Prepare a baking pan or baking sheet. Align it with aluminum foil.

3. Rub and coat the pork with the mixture evenly on all sides. Arrange the pork in the baking pan in single layer and roast for about 45 minutes and until the pork is thoroughly cooked and browned. Wait for 10 minutes before taking the dish out of the oven.

4. Once ready, serve on a platter and garnish with the desired garnishing.

Nutritional Value: Calories – 148; Net Carbs – 1 gram; Protein – 25 grams; Fat – 8 grams

#29 – Vanilla Crème Pudding Parfait

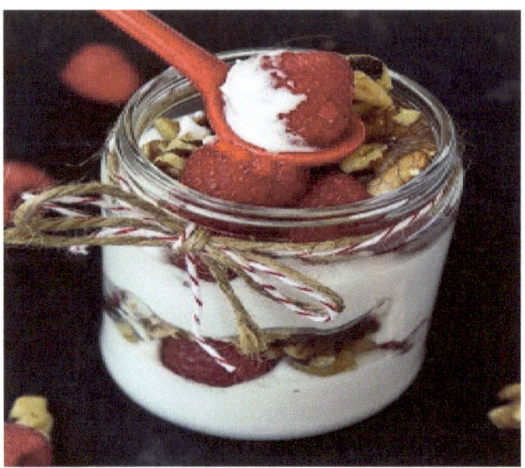

Ingredients

170g of Fresh strawberries

1 can of Full-fat coconut milk, chilled

90g of chopped walnuts

1 tsp. Vanilla extract (pure)

10 drops of Stevia (liquid)

Directions

Combine coconut milk, sweetener, and vanilla extract and thoroughly mix using an electric mixer. Whisk for about 30 seconds until ingredients are well blended. Set aside.

To serve, spoon vanilla crème pudding into half of a glass or jar. Add chopped walnuts and berries and add another layer of the vanilla crème pudding. Sprinkle on top with the remaining walnut and garnish with strawberries.

Nutritional Value: Calories – 399; Net Carbs – 13.1 grams; Protein – 8 grams; Fat – 37.5 grams

#30 – Spicy Jalapeno Poppers

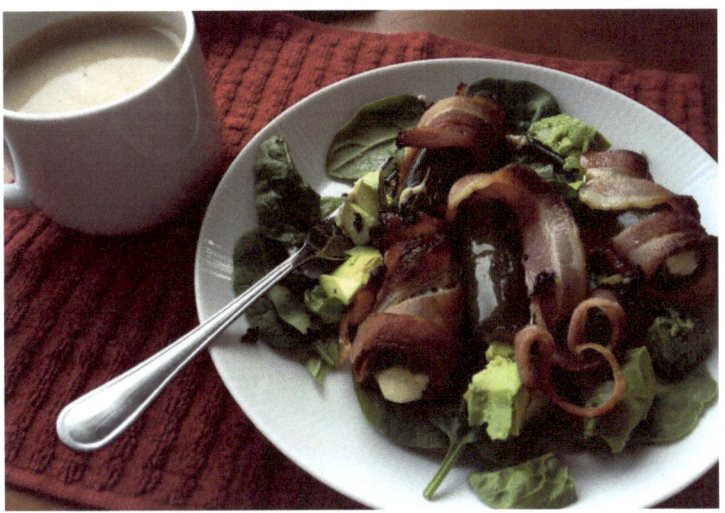

Ingredients

- 12 Bacon slices

- 6 Large jalapenos (Halved and pitted)

- 3 oz. Canned artichokes (Drained and chopped)

- 4 oz. Cream cheese (Cubed)

- 1/4 cup Mayo

- 1 tbsp. White onion (Finely chopped)

- 1/4 cup Pepper Jack Cheese (Shredded)

- 1/4 tsp. Chili powder

- 1/8 tsp. Garlic powder

- Salt

Directions

1. Preheat oven to 400°F.

2. Put artichokes and cream cheese in a large bowl. Microwave for about 30-45 seconds or until the cheese has completely melted. Remove from the microwave and stir.

3. Add cheese, onion, garlic, chili powder, and mayo. Season with salt and mix thoroughly to combine.

4. Put about a tablespoon (or less depending in the size of jalapeno) of artichoke mixture into each jalapeno slice.

5. Wrap each stuffed slice with bacon and arrange them in the baking sheet. Bake for about 30 minutes or until the bacon is crisp and jalapenos are tender. Adjust time according to pepper size and thickness of bacon. Check every 15 minutes to gauge the time needed for cooking.

Nutritional Value: Calories – 146 ; Net Carbs- 2.2 grams; Protein- 5.7 grams; Fat- 11.6 grams